NURTURING WELLNESS WITH IV THERAPY

One Puncture, Countless Miracles to
Recovery and Resilience

Mildred Becky

Table of contents

Introduction

Few inventions in contemporary medicine have captivated the imagination and had such a significant impact on people's lives as intravenous (IV) therapy. This seemingly innocuous medical practice, defined by the mere act of putting a needle into a vein, has grown into a potent tool of wellbeing, particularly for seniors. Its significant influence on health and well-being cannot be emphasized, as it serves as a link between medical knowledge and the human experience, linking one puncture to innumerable miracles and, eventually, supporting recovery and resilience in the golden years.

To begin our trip into the realm of IV Therapy, we must first grasp the foundations. Intravenous Therapy (IV Therapy) is the process of administering fluids, nutrients, drugs, or blood products directly into the bloodstream via a vein. This approach avoids the digestive system, allowing for rapid and effective absorption into the body. While IV Therapy is a flexible medical technique that may be used in a variety of settings, our focus is on its importance for elder wellbeing.

The importance of IV Therapy for seniors arises from its ability to address a wide range of health issues that frequently accompany the aging process. Aging, as a natural process, can cause a variety of physical, emotional, and cognitive changes. Chronic diseases, nutritional deficits, thirst, discomfort, and a variety of other issues may confront seniors. Conventional therapies, while useful, sometimes fall short of providing the prompt and thorough relief that elders desire.

Enter IV Therapy, a fascinating technique that has arisen as a lifeline for elders seeking overall wellbeing rather than simply therapy. It provides a one-of-a-kind confluence of science and compassion, bringing forward the concept that a single puncture can truly result in innumerable miracles in terms of healing and resilience.

Before digging deeper into the wonders it provides, let us first explain how IV Therapy works. Consider a thirsty garden; a conventional watering can represent oral drugs, but a sophisticated irrigation system represents IV Therapy. While both approaches accomplish the same purpose – nurturing the garden – the latter does it with unrivaled efficiency.

The success of intravenous therapy stems on its direct delivery into the bloodstream. When elders get IV treatments, whether water, vitamins, minerals, or prescriptions, these critical chemicals bypass the complicated processes of the digestive system. They quickly enter the circulation, guaranteeing optimum absorption and efficiency. Because of this distinguishing feature, IV Therapy is especially advantageous for elderly, who may have damaged digestive systems or difficulties absorbing nutrition adequately.

The route from one puncture to innumerable miracles begins with thorough planning and an awareness of the patient's unique requirements. Seniors who receive IV Therapy go on a path that is individualized to their specific health state and needs.

The IV Therapy method is proof of current medical accuracy. Trained healthcare experts undertake a step-by-step procedure, from finding the best vein to giving the therapy at the appropriate rate. Monitoring vital indicators and keeping sterile conditions are critical safety considerations.

Seniors frequently see instant improvements as the IV infusion develops. Dehydration is quickly eased, which is a significant problem among seniors owing to factors such as decreasing fluid consumption or medicines. Nutritional deficiencies that might cause weariness, weakness, and cognitive impairment are treated as soon as possible. Furthermore, IV Therapy relieves pain effectively, making it a vital tool in the management of illnesses such as arthritis, fibromyalgia, and even post-surgery discomfort.

The wonders weaved within IV Therapy are arguably most visible when evaluating the specific illnesses and disorders it tackles. Seniors suffering from chronic conditions such as diabetes, COPD, or heart disease find refuge in the regular respite and symptom control that IV Therapy provides.

Furthermore, IV Therapy has shown to be quite useful in the management of acute health problems. Seniors suffering from severe infections, acute dehydration, or the after effects of chemotherapy frequently see significant improvement in their illnesses. It is very unusual for IV Therapy to be the tipping point in their recovery journey, transforming them from despair to optimism.

Clinical proof and real-life success stories attest to the marvels that IV Therapy may do. Seniors who have had IV treatments commonly describe their life-changing experiences. These tales act as beacons of hope for others, motivating them to look into IV Therapy as a way to improve their quality of life and speed up their recovery.

Beyond its immediate therapeutic effects, IV Therapy is critical in cultivating resilience in seniors. This resilience includes both bodily and emotional well-being.

Long-term wellbeing is a priority. Seniors are increasingly resorting to preventive IV Therapy to remain on top of their health. IV Therapy becomes a proactive tool for aging gracefully by correcting vitamin shortages, boosting the immune system, and improving general vitality.

However, the advantages go well beyond the physical sphere. IV Therapy recognizes the deep relationship between mind and body. Seniors who receive IV treatments frequently report improved mood, cognitive performance, and emotional well-being. Physical discomfort relief can reduce tension and anxiety, contributing to an improved overall quality of life.

IV Therapy is a revolutionary path for seniors, leading from one puncture to many miracles while building healing and resilience. As we delve deeper into the world of IV Therapy, we'll look at not only its benefits, but also the safety concerns, the promising future it holds in senior healthcare, and the collective responsibility we all bear in ensuring that this invaluable tool continues to enrich the lives of our aging population. Join us as we explore the wonders of IV Therapy, including its ability to reignite hope, regenerate bodies, and revive souls in our golden years.

Chapter 1: Understanding IV Therapy

The injection of nutrients and water directly into the circulation for prompt absorption and usage by the body is known as IV therapy, sometimes known as intravenous therapy.

Because it skips the digestive system and goes directly into the organs, IV Therapy is the quickest way to transport nutrients throughout the body, resulting in a 90-100% absorption rate (as compared to only 20-50% orally).

With one-third of UK employees suffering from anxiety, depression, or stress (according to a PwC poll), it's no surprise that there's a rising need for preventative and therapeutic IV vitamin clinics that can increase energy levels and activate the immune system.

Although the media depicts IV Therapy as the latest health trend popular among stressed-out city workers, sportsmen, and Hollywood celebrities, the technique has been around for decades.

An Overview of IV Therapy

IV therapy is not a novel medical treatment, nor is it a passing trend. In the 1600s, medical practitioners attempted to inject drugs into veins, but the technique was abandoned due to inadequate cleanliness.

IV Therapy became a lifesaving treatment during World War I, but it wasn't until the 1960s, when Dr. John Myers produced a world-famous mixture of vitamins and minerals, that the intravenous vitamin therapy we know today began to take shape.

What Is the Purpose of IV Therapies?

IV treatment is used for a variety of reasons, including:

→ Recovery from a hangover.
→ Athletic performance recuperation.
→ Immunity boosting.
→ Cold and flu treatment.
→ Inflammation.
→ Problems with digestion.

→ Exhaustion.

→ Improved sleep patterns due to blood sugar balance.

→ Migraines are less common.

→ Fertility enhancement and hormonal imbalance.

→ improved skin tone.

Who Is a Candidate for IV Therapy?

Intravenous nutrients were originally used mostly in hospitals for patients who were dehydrated, nutrient-deficient, or unable to take prescriptions orally.

IV Vitamin Therapy can now help people who are in good health improve their wellbeing and energy levels.

The stress of contemporary life may deplete your immune system and overall well-being; IV Therapy can provide that much-needed boost, making it a realistic and practical solution.

While stress does not cause us to develop a cold or flu virus, it can reduce our immune system's capacity to respond to viruses, making us more susceptible to infection and sickness.

If you want to enhance your immunity, replace lost fluids and electrolytes after a night of drinking, or promote recovery from high-performance athletics, IV Vitamin Therapy can assist.

The most common reason people seek treatment from us is stress. The Myers Cocktail IV and Immunity Booster IV treatments are popular with our customers who want to feel energized and increase their immunity.

What Is the IV Therapy Procedure?

Even though IV treatment requires inserting a needle into the arm or other parts of the body, the little discomfort is felt only when the skin is initially penetrated.

All clients' medical histories are reviewed prior to therapy. A blood test is performed if necessary to ensure that the proper amount of nutrients are pumped into the body.

After the consultation, you will be taken to our light IV Therapy room and situated in a comfortable chair to begin the treatment. The rate and amount of intravenous fluid supplied to each customer is determined by their medical condition, weight, and age.

After disinfecting the skin above the injection site, which is usually on your arm, a competent doctor or nurse will find a vein and install an IV catheter.

The operation will take between 15 and 45 minutes once the catheter is in place, depending on the kind of treatment (IV Drip or IV Push).

The only thing you need to do at this time is rest. You can watch television, read a magazine, or even take a sleep.

Do you want to know how IV drips can help you? Here's all you need to know about IV treatment kinds.

If you wish to enhance your health or have a more beautiful complexion, IV treatment can assist. Throughout the therapy, vitamins and minerals are directly infused into your bloodstream to give you more radiant skin. Each IV drip contains a unique blend of antioxidants, electrolytes, vital fluids, and vitamins.

What distinguishes IV drips from supplements, and why are they so effective? In contrast to supplements, which must be broken down before the body can absorb them, important vitamins and minerals are injected intravenously into the system. As a result, IV treatment considerably accelerates the process of resupplying the body with critical vitamins and minerals.

What are the many forms of IV therapy?

Here are some examples of popular IV therapies:

IV INFUSION DETOXIFICATION BOOSTER

Did you know that a buildup of toxins in fat cells makes it difficult to lose weight? This drip contains important fluids, vitamins, and minerals that can help with toxic load reduction.

IV THERAPY TO BOOST IMMUNITY

This IV treatment uses a robust antioxidant combination such as glutathione, cysteine, and arginine to help protect you from the flu and other illnesses.

IV MYERS COCKTAIL THERAPY

This magnesium, B vitamin, and vitamin C infusion helps treat a range of ailments, including fatigue and poor immunity.

HYDRATION IV DRIP

IV hydration treatment benefits persons who have lost fluids as a result of vomiting, diarrhea, or hangovers, as well as athletes who want to perform at their peak.

IV NAD+ ANTI-AGING THERAPY

This comprises nicotinamide adenine dinucleotide (NAD+), an enzyme found in all human cells. Its two primary benefits are cell healing and lowering the body's oxidative stress.

What are the advantages of receiving IV drips?

IV drips provide several skin and health advantages, including:

SKIN WITH LUMINOUS SKIN

Did you realize that your skin affects your health? A functioning liver, for example, is necessary for healthy skin. Similarly, a lack of certain nutrients can cause your skin to seem dull and lifeless. IV drips provide a variety of critical minerals such as magnesium and zinc, as well as B-complex vitamins and vitamin C, all of which support good skin function. Glutathione, a potent antioxidant, is given intravenously to assist your liver and kidneys in cleansing. As a consequence, your skin appears attractive and youthful.

BODY HYDRATED

If you're having difficulties staying hydrated, IV drips are an excellent option. Electrolytes, in addition to replenishing our bodies, control blood pressure, neuron and muscle activity, and other physiological activities. Your body need electrolytes such as potassium, calcium, bicarbonate, magnesium, chloride, phosphate, and sodium. These electrolytes are administered by IV infusions to replenish your body and keep you competitive.

PROTECTION OF THE IMMUNE SYSTEM

IV drips provide health-improving nutrients directly into your circulation. As a result, they are a wonderful method to enhance your immune system. Routine IV infusions can protect you against a variety of ailments.

IV INfusions for **IMPROVED attention** make you feel better physically and emotionally, reduce tension and anxiety, and increase your attention. They can also increase dopamine and serotonin levels, which can improve your mood.

REVIVAL OF JET LAG

IV drips are especially useful for frequent travelers since they assist to battle jet lag caused by dehydration and electrolyte imbalance during flight.

DETOXIFICATION

IV drips are a highly effective detoxification therapy. By infusing critical nutrients and trace elements into the bloodstream, the process assists in the efficient elimination of pollutants and toxins from the body, detoxing and purifying your blood.

If you desire clear, healthy skin or better general health, try Biolite's customized IV drips. Our staff meticulously evaluates your medical history and goals in order to build an IV drip that exactly addresses your difficulties.

The two main types of IV therapy

IV Therapy is classified into two types: IV Push and IV Drip.

The key distinctions are the duration of the therapy and the volume of fluid infused.

Vitamin absorption is 90-100% with both IV Push and IV Drip therapies.

What Exactly Is An IV Drip?

An IV drip is a form of intravenous therapy in which medication is slowly administered into the circulation using a plastic catheter put into a vein.

To administer an IV Drip, a needle is used to put a tiny plastic tube (catheter) into a vein, which is then swiftly withdrawn once the plastic tube is progressed into the vein.

IV drips last 45-60 minutes, with an average of 250-1000 cc of fluid delivered every session.

Clients can read, work, or rest while on a drip.

What Exactly Is An IV Push?

An IV Push is administered gently into a vein using a previously placed plastic catheter.

IV pushes last 15-20 minutes, and a total of 30-60 cc of fluid is progressively pumped into a vein.

Because of the nature of the procedure, IV Pushes are always overseen by professionals.

Depending on the therapy, the ingredients of an IV drip will differ. Because an IV drip is the fastest means to deliver fluids and drugs into the bloodstream, it is often composed of the following:

Saline solution: A sterile solution of water and salt used to hydrate the body and maintain electrolyte balance.

A sterile solution of water and glucose (sugar) that supplies energy to the organism.

IV drips can also contain nutrients such as vitamins, minerals, and amino acids, which are necessary for the body to operate correctly.

When admitted to the hospital, the IV drip may appear a little different. While it may still contain the fluids described above, it may additionally contain:

drugs: Depending on the illness being treated, different drugs might be mixed into the IV drip to alleviate pain, nausea, infection, or other medical conditions.

Blood products: In some situations, IV drips may be used to replenish factors such as red blood cells, plasma, or platelets in order to treat problems such as anemia or bleeding disorders, or if the patient has been harmed and lost blood.

Contrast agents: Substances used in medical imaging to make specific structures or fluids in the body more visible. They are sometimes administered by IV drip during imaging procedures such as CT scans or MRIs.

In IV Therapy, what vitamin cocktails are used?

Vitamin C, B vitamins, magnesium, calcium, and zinc are all common constituents in IV vitamin treatment.

IV vitamin drips can also include amino acids and antioxidants like glutathione.

Vitamin infusions can be made up of a single vitamin, such as vitamin C, or a combination of vitamins and minerals.

What Are the Most Frequently Used IV Vitamin Cocktail Drips?

Myers Cocktail IV - This drip, which contains magnesium, B vitamins, and vitamin C, is said to cure a variety of medical issues, including immunity and energy levels.

Hydration IV Drip - IV hydration therapy aids patients recuperating from fluid loss due to vomiting, diarrhea, or a hangover, as well as athletes looking to improve their performance.

IV NAD+ Anti-Aging Therapy - This comprises nicotinamide adenine dinucleotide (NAD+), an enzyme found in all human cells. Its major job is to repair damaged cells and counteract oxidative stress in the body.

Detoxification Booster IV Infusion - A drip containing critical fluids, vitamins, and minerals that have been shown to reduce toxic load. Toxins are accumulated in fat cells, making weight loss more difficult.

Immunity Booster IV - A mixture of potent antioxidants such as glutathione, cysteine, and arginine that aids in the prevention of flu and other viruses.

How long do the effects of IV therapy last?

Although many patients report feeling better shortly after treatment, the benefits usually become completely apparent 12 - 24 hours following infusion.

Depending on the disease, cocktail, and kind of IV Therapy, the effects might range from 8 days to 3 weeks.

Is IV Therapy Risky?

Today, intravenous fluid delivery by IV infusion is widespread and typically safe, but having too much of a good thing might raise the chance of unwanted consequences.

If you have a medical problem, it is always best to contact with your doctor before beginning any therapy to avoid consequences.

There is also a danger of infection due to the penetration of your skin. Although the chance of skin or blood infection is remote, it is important to seek the advice of a skilled medical practitioner to guarantee a safe and healthy vitamin infusion.

Important Considerations When Planning IV Therapy

If you have a specific medical problem, consult with your primary care physician to see if IV Vitamin Therapy is correct for you.

Make certain that the doctor from whom you are having IV vitamin treatment is certified and is aware of all of your health ailments and concerns.

It is critical that you conduct research about the clinic before scheduling an appointment. Before approving you for the treatment, the licensed clinic should conduct a complete medical examination.

Clinicians must inquire about your medical history, medicines, and allergies before deciding whether to reject or appoint you.

You should never feel rushed, and a nurse should always explain what is happening to you. When in doubt, never be scared to request credentials. Choose your clinic carefully!

Chapter 2: How IV Therapy works

In medicine, intravenous (or IV) refers to the delivery of drugs into the body via a vein or veins. IV treatment works by injecting fluids straight into your veins. There are two main types of IV therapy:

1. Infusion

A syringe is used to drive a liquid into the body during injection. IV injection is the quickest delivery technique and gives the most immediate results of all injection modalities (described below). In addition to intravenous administration, injections can be administered by a variety of methods, including:

Intradermal injections are administered directly into the dermis (the skin's main layer). This injection type has the slowest absorption rate among the injectable kinds and is typically used for sensitivity assessments.

Intramuscular (IM) injections are administered deep into a muscle and rapidly absorbed by blood vessels. Flu shots and epi-pens, for example, are frequently administered in the thigh, shoulder, or buttock.

Subcutaneous (SubQ) injections are administered at the skin's deepest layer. These injections are slower than intramuscular injections but faster than intradermal injections. Subcutaneous injections are often used for PROCRIT, Aranesp, RETACRITTM, Prolia, XOLAIR, and NUCALA.

While injection is the most prevalent method of intravenous administration, when most people refer to "an IV," they are referring to the second type of IV therapy, infusion.

2. injection

Infusion, as opposed to injection, employs a pump or the natural force of gravity to transfer fluids into the body. As a result, they are frequently referred to as drips. The purpose of an IV infusion is to infuse a chemical into the circulation in a regulated manner over time. Infusion periods will differ depending on what is a safe drip rate for a particular drug or supplement.

A bag with the substance being supplied is suspended from a pole, and lines are sent to a catheter in the patient's vein, which is most typically placed in the wrist, elbow, or back of hand. IV infusions, like IV injections, deliver medication directly into the circulation, resulting in faster absorption and more obvious instant effects. Some infusion therapies are administered through the skin and muscles, but IV infusion is the most common type of infusion therapy available today.

Getting to Your Vein

Our nurses insert a catheter, which is a little, thin plastic tube, directly into your vein. To assist reduce any discomfort, we utilize a numbing spray when inserting the catheter.

Taking Out the Needle

We remove the needle when our nurse has accessed your vein. The catheter is left within while you provide your IV infusion.

Putting the Drip Bag Together

The catheter is connected to a bag that carries your chosen drip!

Sit back, relax, and take it all in.

An IV drip takes around 30 to 45 minutes to complete a whole therapy session, including the initial paperwork.

What is in an IV?

Electrolytes and salts are found in certain IV drips, whereas carbohydrates, vitamins, and antioxidants are found in others. Each combination is unique to the patient's health and wellbeing demands.

The following are the most frequent substances found in IVs:

The most common form of fluid for IVs is saline, which is a salt solution in water. Because sodium is an electrolyte, a saline solution is excellent for dehydration and hangovers.

Vitamins and antioxidants are important since they may give us greater energy, enhance our immune system, and do so much more.

Electrolytes are vital components and compounds that hydrate our bodies, regulate neuron and muscle function, and control blood pressure, among other things. In addition to sodium, your body need potassium, calcium, bicarbonate, magnesium, chloride, and phosphate, which are all electrolytes.

Bounce Hydration can include a variety of different substances in addition to these usual ones. For example, we provide anti-nausea and anti-inflammatory medications, both of which are widely used to treat hangover symptoms.

As a drip hydration treatment spa, we employ all of these substances to create drips based on our patients' wellbeing needs. Some IVs, such as our Fit Drip, are intended to assist weight reduction and contain a metabolism stimulant. Others, such as our Revitalizing Drip, are intended to alleviate the long-term consequences of diseases, such as Covid-19, and our Immunity Warrior

Drip, which is meant to combat viruses, germs, and seasonal allergens.

Value in Senior Healthcare

When it comes to the vitamins and nutrients our systems require to function optimally, the fact is that we don't always get all we need from meals and oral supplements.

This is where IV nutritional treatment can help. This type of therapy, which is intended to supplement a healthy diet and active lifestyle, may provide a range of advantages, ranging from increasing recovery time after an accident to helping improve your immune system.

Is IV Nutritional Therapy Safe for Seniors?

One common misperception concerning IV nutritional treatment is that it is only appropriate for adolescents. But that is not the case! Adults of all ages can benefit from the numerous IV vitamin treatment benefits. Here are some of the advantages that older persons may gain from IV nutritional treatment.

Benefit #1: IV vitamin treatment can help you feel better overall.

The advantages of IV vitamin treatment might range from fewer headaches and enhanced immunity to reduced anxiety and a number of other benefits. Many individuals elect to receive IV nutritional treatment in order to enhance their immune systems.

Maintaining a robust immune system is more critical than ever for older persons and people with significant underlying medical disorders. Learn more about Olympia Compounding Pharmacy's Immunity IV Kit and how it may help boost your immune system right now.

Benefit #2: IV vitamin treatment works swiftly.

Another significant advantage of IV vitamin therapy is that you may begin to feel the results almost immediately. Other vitamin-enriched drugs and foods must pass through the digestive system and may take some time to absorb into the body. Because IV vitamin treatment is administered intravenously, it enters the circulation immediately, allowing nutrients to be absorbed quickly.

Benefit #3: It can assist in healthy weight loss.

Losing weight may be difficult for everyone. However, losing weight can be especially difficult for older persons as metabolisms slow and muscle mass begins to decline—even for those who stay physically active.

IV nutritional treatment can aid in weight reduction in several ways:

Hydration is an important aspect in weight reduction since it increases metabolism, inhibits hunger, and cleanses the body of toxins. Discover how our Quench IV Kit may help you rehydrate, cleanse, and replenish vital vitamins.

Sleep deprivation has been linked to weight growth on several occasions. Lack of sleep was a key issue that hindered some people from losing weight even when they followed a rigorous diet and exercised often. Adults should sleep between 7-9 hours every night, depending on their particular demands.

Vitamin Absorption: As previously said, when the body is able to absorb nutrients completely through the bloodstream, it is obtaining what it requires to work optimally. When you can recover faster after an exercise, you may start the following session earlier and push harder, which helps to speed up your metabolism and promote weight loss.

Benefit #4: It may aid in the reduction of the effects of aging.

IV vitamin treatment can also assist to cool the skin from within. At Olympia, we have an IV kit called Inner Beauty that is specifically created for bringing out your skin's natural shine, eliminating wrinkles, and making your skin seem beautiful. It contains ascorbic acid, B-complex vitamins, and biotin, all of which are necessary elements for keeping healthy skin and blood cells.

Benefit #5: It can provide a source of energy.

Low B12 levels, stress, lack of sleep, electrolyte imbalances, and other factors can all contribute to a lack of energy. IV drips assist counteract these concerns since they are high in important vitamins and nutrients, reducing the need for additional (sometimes harmful) energy supplements such as coffee, energy drinks, cola, and so on. One important advantage of IV vitamin treatment is that it can help combat fatigue and increase circulation, therefore enhancing your overall energy levels and metabolism.

Chapter 3: The Process: From Puncture to Miracles

A. BASICS OF IV THERAPY

Infusion of Primary IV Fluids

Primary IV fluid infusions are used by doctors to restore or maintain hydration and electrolyte balance in the body. When delivering IV fluids to a patient, the nurse must constantly check the patient's fluid and electrolyte status in order to assess the efficacy of the infusion and avoid potential problems of fluid excess and electrolyte imbalance.

The most frequent primary IV fluid bag holds 1,000 mL. Bags are also available in 500 mL, 250 mL, 100 mL, and 50 mL sizes. The primary fluid bag size is determined by infusion requirement, patient condition, and age. Because of the greater drip (gtt) rate, most adult patients get continuous IV fluids in 1,000 mL bags. For intermittent infusions or short-term treatment, several additional fluid volume bags are employed.

For example, because high quantities of continuous fluids are contraindicated in renal dialysis patients due to their renal impairment, IV bags less than 1,000 mL are utilized. Many hospitals may display lower capacity normal saline continuous infusion bags as a warning that these patients should not get huge volumes of main fluids. Pediatric patients, who, due to their lesser anatomical size, do not require significant main fluid infusion volumes, are another example of patients that require smaller IV bags.

An IV pump is primarily used to give primary fluids. An IV pump is the most secure way to ensuring that specified volumes of fluid are delivered. However, there may be times when IV pumps are not accessible and nurses must provide main fluids through drip tube by gravity. In the "Math Calculation" chapter, you may learn more about determining infusion rates.

Primary fluids are infused at regular rates for a set amount of time. For example, a continuous fluid infusion of 125 mL/hour for 24 hours may be scheduled. Continuous fluids may also be ordered to run until the provider issues a further order to stop or reduce the fluid rate.

IV primary fluid bags include a variety of fluids, including 0.9% normal saline, 0.45% (12) normal saline, lactated ringers solution, and dextrose (5%). They may also contain electrolytes such as potassium chloride as replacements. Primary fluids will be ordered by the clinician depending on the patient's fluid and electrolyte state.

Intravenous fluid concentrations are classified as isotonic, hypertonic, or hypotonic.

Isotonic fluids are commonly used to replenish fluid and electrolytes. Because isotonic fluids have a comparable concentration to the solutes found in blood, they do not trigger osmotic fluid movement into or out of the patient's individual cells. 0.9% normal saline is an example of isotonic fluid.

Solute concentrations in hypertonic fluids are greater than in blood. They are commonly used in critical care circumstances to treat hyponatremia and prevent pulmonary edema by relying on osmosis to eliminate excess fluid. Dextrose 5% in 0.9% normal saline (D5NS) is an example of a hypertonic fluid.

Solute concentrations in hypotonic fluids are lower than in blood. The purpose of hypotonic fluid administration is to transfer fluids into the cells of a patient by osmosis. When a patient has severe intracellular dehydration, such as diabetic ketoacidosis, hypotonic treatments are routinely employed. Hypotonic fluid is defined as 0.45% normal saline (1/2NS). Figure 23.1[1] depicts the effects of hypertonic, isotonic, and hypotonic IV fluid delivery on a patient's red blood cells.

Because a patient's fluid and electrolyte statuses are continually changing when getting IV fluids, it is critical for the nurse to watch for indicators of fluid or electrolyte imbalances and contact the health care provider as soon as possible. When a patient is getting nothing by mouth (NPO), for example, primary fluids may be begun at a greater rate of infusion, but should be decreased when they resume regular food and fluid consumption. To provide essential insight into a patient's fluid volume status, the nurse must constantly evaluate their skin turgor, urine output, lung sounds, and oxygen requirements, as well as screen for any new edema. A nurse must also assess the effects of replacement fluids and consult with the prescribing practitioner about their continued requirement.

Infusion of Secondary Fluids

Secondary IV fluid delivery is often performed as an intermittent infusion at regular intervals (e.g., every 8 hours). This type of IV treatment often includes drugs delivered in a smaller infusion bag and combined with a diluent fluid such as saline (e.g., IV antibiotics). Many typical preparations are available in 25-100 mL bags.

Because it is linked to the principal bag of intravenous fluids, secondary IV treatment is sometimes known as "IV piggyback" (IVPB) medicine. The primary line in this example preserves venous access between medication dosages.

It is vital to realize that not all IV fluids and drugs are compatible. The nurse must triple-check that the secondary medications/fluids are compatible with the primary fluids. If the drug and fluids are incompatible, a precipitate may develop when the fluids mix within the line, endangering the patient's health.

IV Administration Supplies

Intravenous (IV) fluids and drugs are delivered using a flexible plastic tubing system known as an IV administration set. The IV administration set attaches the solution bag to the patient's IV access site. Primary tubing and secondary tubing are the two main types of IV administration systems. Furthermore, IV fluids can be supplied by gravity or by infusion pump, each with its own administration set.

Sets for Primary IV Administration

Primary IV administration settings are used to infuse fluids or drugs continuously or intermittently. A macro-drip or micro-drip solution set can be used for primary IV tubing. A macro-drip infusion set produces 10, 15, or 20 drops per milliliter, whereas a micro-drip infusion set produces 60 drops per milliliter. The drop factor is printed on the IV tubing package and must be verified when determining medicine delivery rates. Adults employ macro-drip sets for routine primary infusions. Micro-drip IV tubing is used in pediatric or newborn care to provide little volumes of fluids over a lengthy period of time.

The following items are included in primary IV administration sets:

Sterile spike: As you spike the IV fluid bag, this component of the tubing must be maintained sterile.

Drip chamber: A drip chamber allows air to rise from a fluid and not be transmitted onto the patient. It is also used to compute the rate of fluid administration by gravity (drops per minute). Keep it 14 to 12 full of solution.

A backcheck valve prevents fluid or medicines from ascending into the primary IV bag.

Access ports are utilized to infuse secondary drugs as well as to provide IV push medications. These are sometimes referred to as "Y ports."

Roller clamp: A roller clamp is used to slow or halt an infusion via gravity.

Sets of Secondary Iv Administration

Secondary IV administration sets are used to provide a secondary drug, such as an antibiotic, sporadically while the original IV is still running. Secondary IV tubing is shorter than primary tubing and connects to a primary line through an access port or an IV pump. The secondary infusion is attached to an access port and suspended above the original infusion.

To ensure that the right amount of medication is given, secondary fluids should always be "piggybacked" into primary infusion lines. The solution from the primary fluid line is utilized to prime the secondary tubing by piggybacking a medicine. However, if a secondary infusion is used as a main fluid, part of the secondary medicine may be lost upon priming the line, resulting in less medication being delivered. Medication loss is classified as a medication mistake since the patient received less active medicine than was recommended.

Administration of IV fluids

When starting or changing an IV bag of fluids or drugs, keep the following factors in mind:

IV fluids are a type of medicine. Verify doctors orders and ensure the patient is not allergic to this drug. Perform the six drug administration rights three times, just as you would with any other medicine. Check the fluid kind and expiry date, and make sure it's free of discolouration and sediment. When purchasing a new tubing administration set, make sure to check the expiration date.

Examine the bag to check that it is not leaking and is not damaged. It is common for moisture to accumulate on the interior of the plastic IV bag storage container.

Check that the IV fluid infusion rate is suitable for the patient's age, size, prior medical problems, and recommended indication. If a manual calculation is required to establish the IV flow rate, perform the computation and double-check the result with another registered nurse.

To avoid infection, IV tube administration sets must be replaced on a regular basis. Before starting a new bag of fluids or drugs, follow agency policy about tube changes.

If there is administration set tubing present, trace it from the patient to its point of origin to ensure that you are accessing the proper port.

Examine the IV area. Examine for redness, swelling, or discomfort, which might indicate irritation, inflammation, or infection.

When starting a new fluid or medicine, make sure the IV site is patent. As per agency protocol, aspirate for blood return and flush the IV catheter.

The Risks of IV Therapy

It is critical to screen for potential problems such as infiltration, extravasation, phlebitis, or infection while monitoring a patient receiving IV fluids. If any of these issues arise, contact your provider immediately for treatment; the IV catheter may need to be withdrawn and replaced at a different location, and more medicine may be recommended.

Infiltration happens when the catheter tip falls out of the vein. The catheter penetrates through the vein wall or the blood vessel wall, allowing some of the fluid to infuse into the surrounding tissue, resulting in IV fluid leakage into the surrounding tissue. Infiltration can result in discomfort, edema, and cool-to-the-touch skin. If you suspect an IV has been tampered with, follow your facility's guidelines and, as a general rule, cease the site and transfer the IV. If the infiltration is extensive, you should use a compress in addition to elevating the afflicted leg. Check your institution's policy to see if a warm or cold compress should be used.[4],[5] Clinical pharmacists can also be valuable resources for choosing the best type of infiltration therapy.

Extravasation is the infiltration of harmful intravenous drugs, such as chemotherapy, into the extravascular tissue around the infusion site. Extravasation causes tissue harm and, depending on the medicine, location, and time of exposure, tissue death, also known as necrosis. Extravasation can be treated with drugs that help avoid the complication of necrosis if caught early.

Phlebitis is a vein irritation: Phlebitis of superficial veins can arise as a result of damage to the vein after IV catheter placement. If not treated properly, it can cause redness and pain around the vein and lead to infection. Warm compresses and nonsteroidal anti-inflammatory medicines may be used to treat the condition.

When the skin barrier is disrupted by inserting an IV catheter, infection might arise. Infection symptoms include redness, warmth, soreness, and even fever. Vascular catheter-associated infection is classified as a hospital-acquired illness since it is avoidable by following best practices. To reduce the risk of vascular catheter-associated infection, use evidence-based infection prevention practices such as hand hygiene, a vigorous mechanical scrub of needleless connectors, limiting catheter access, and using a sterile no-touch technique during intravenous infusion.

The nurse should collect critical subjective and objective evaluation information from the patient in order to prepare for intravenous treatment delivery.

Subjective Evaluation

When doing the subjective evaluation, the nurse should start by collecting facts that might indicate a potential problem if the patient receives IV infusion treatment. The nurse should start by determining whether the patient has any pharmaceutical allergies or a latex allergy. The patient's history should also be evaluated, with specific consideration given to individuals with known congestive heart failure (CHF) or chronic kidney disease (CKD), as they are more prone to fluid overload. Furthermore, the patient should be questioned whether they are experiencing any pain or discomfort at their IV access site now or throughout the medicine or fluid infusion.

Considerations Regarding Life Expectancy

Special patient populations' needs and characteristics, such as physiologic, developmental, communication/cognitive ability, and/or safety requirements, are identified and addressed during the planning, insertion, removal, care, management, and monitoring of vascular access devices (VADs) and infusion therapy administration.

Children's safety measures for an IV infusion include checking the IV site for patency every hour. According to agency policy, infused amounts and indications of fluid excess should be thoroughly examined and documented on a regular basis.

To prevent the youngster from messing with the IV site or tubing, joint stabilization may be used. It should, however, be used in a fashion that allows for visual examination and assessment of the vascular access site and the vascular pathway, and it should not impose pressure that causes circulatory constriction, pressure injury, or nerve damage in the region of flexion or under the device. It should also be removed on a regular basis to examine vascular health, range of motion and function, and skin integrity. Due to the danger of fungal infection, wooden tongue depressors should not be utilized as joint stabilization devices in premature newborns or immunocompromised adults.

Furthermore, the tubing should be well-secured, and the dressing should be kept dry so that the IV site is not compromised. Be mindful that mobile youngsters will require supervision to ensure that the tubing is not clogged if they unintentionally sit or sleep on it.

Senior Citizens

Nurses must identify physiologic changes associated with aging and their impact on immunity, medication dose and volume restrictions, pharmacologic activities, interactions, side effects, monitoring parameters, and infusion treatment response. Anatomical alterations, such as loss of dermal skin layer thickness, thickening of the tunica intima/media, and loss of connective tissue, all contribute to vein fragility and provide difficulties in vascular access. Nurses must examine any changes in cognitive capacities, dexterity, and the capacity to communicate or learn that may affect IV treatment (e.g., changes in vision, hearing, or speech).

Fluid volume overload in older persons receiving IV infusions should be checked on a regular basis. Elevated blood pressure and respiratory rate, reduced oxygen saturation, peripheral edema, small crackles in the posterior lower lobes of the lungs, and evidence of increasing heart failure are all symptoms of fluid volume overload. Furthermore, elderly persons have fragile venous walls that may not be able to resist fast infusion rates. When infusing large volumes of fluids at quicker rates, it is critical to closely check the IV site patency and adjust the infusion rate as needed.

A stethoscope image in a circleAssess the IV site for symptoms of problems every time you engage with the patient, and instruct the patient to notify you if there is soreness or swelling at the IV site.

Objective Evaluation

Follow the agency's IV treatment assessment and documentation policies and procedures. Current infusion standards recommend that the venous access device site, the entire infusion system, and the patient be evaluated for signs of complications on a regular basis, depending on a number of factors such as the patient's age, condition, and cognition; the type and frequency of intravenous fluid/medication; and the health care setting. Peripherally inserted IVs should be assessed at least every 4 hours in inpatient and nursing facilities, with increased frequency of assessment every 1 to 2 hours for patients who are critically ill, sedated, or have cognitive deficits, and hourly for neonatal/pediatric patients and patients receiving vesicant medication infusions.

Throughout the course of therapy, the nurse routinely assesses the complete IV infusion system, from the patient's IV insertion site and dressing to the IV solution container, for system integrity, infusion accuracy, detection of problems, and expiration dates. Redness, pallor, swelling, coldness, or warmth to the touch should be absent from the IV site, and the IV infusion should flow easily.

The nurse should also be familiar with the various forms of intravenous access that might be utilized for an infusion. A peripherally inserted central catheter (PICC), for example, resembles intravenous access but requires different evaluation and monitoring than a central line.

B. The IV Therapy Procedure

It is critical to inspect the fluid bag before starting an intravenous fluid infusion. Despite the fact that the fluids are different, the bags all have the same construction and labeling.

→ The kind of fluid
→ Fluid expiration date
→ Injection point
→ Insertion port for providing spike

Procedures

Introduce yourself to the patient, review the patient's information, and review the prescription sheet. Take note of the fluid type, volume, and time allotted. Make cautious to rule out any allergies.

Inform the patient about the operation and obtain their permission. Check the fluid bag for cloudiness or particle matter; if such contaminants are present, do not use the bag. Remove the bag's outer wrapping and hang it on a drip stand.

Using the roller-ball clamp on the line, open the giving set and close the flow control. By twisting and tearing it off, remove the lid from the port on the bag. Insert the spike without contacting the end into the port.

Squeeze the filling chamber halfway, then release the roller ball clamp to let the fluid to flow through the giving set. Check for bubbles in the line and remove the roller ball.

Put on an apron and gloves to protect your hands. Clean the bionector hub with a chlorhexidine wipe before flushing the cannula with saline. Connect the bionector to the providing set. Adjust the roller ball to set the infusion rate.

Drip Rate Calculation

The drip rate is the number of fluid droplets that enter the filling chamber per minute. The drip rate is manually adjusted and controls how quickly the fluid is administered into the patient. It is determined as follows:

First, determine the needed ml/hr:

For example, a 1 litre bag of normal saline delivered over 8 hours = 1000ml/8hrs = 125ml/hr
Then compute the needed ml/min:

For example, 125ml/hr = 125ml/60mins = 2ml/min
20 drops in 1ml for a normal gifting set. As a result, you can compute the number of droplets per minute as follows:

2mls/min = 40 drops/min, for example.

How IV Therapy Can Aid in the Treatment of Chronic Pain

Chronic pain can arise for a variety of causes. An sickness or accident can cause long-term nerve damage in certain persons. Sometimes there is inflammation that does not improve with time. Chronic pain has an influence on your day-to-day life. Even if you've tried everything else, there is a therapy that may assist. Many people can benefit from IV treatment to achieve the relief they want.

Living with chronic pain not only has an influence on your quality of life, but it can also shorten your life. Due to inactivity, men and women with this illness are frequently overweight. They may have health issues such as heart disease or diabetes. Many have limitations that limit their ability to perform things they like, which often leads to depression. Many individuals are unaware that there are therapeutic alternatives other than pain drugs that can assist with chronic ailments like these.

The purpose of IV treatment is to feed the body with a high amount of excellent nourishment. IV treatment nutrients may include magnesium, calcium, Vitamin C, and B vitamins. These nutrients can aid to increase several of the organ's functions, such as immune system stimulation. It also aids the body in its battle against inflammation and damage.

A person receives an increased amount of vitamins and minerals via an intravenous line during IV treatment. The nutrients do not pass via the digestive system because they enter the bloodstream. That implies the nutrients are more complete and easily absorbed by the cells. The entire procedure takes under an hour. There is some time to relax throughout the therapy. Most people have little discomfort and are able to resume their normal activities immediately.

How does this help with your pain?

IV treatment is tailored to your unique requirements. To do this, your doctors will collaborate with you to determine the source of your discomfort. If inflammation is present, for example, the appropriate IV therapy will try to stimulate your immune system, urging it to repair these places and minimize the inflammation. In certain circumstances, muscular injury may occur. An injection of magnesium or other minerals can aid in the regeneration of these regions.

Why should IV treatment be preferred over pain medications?

Many people use pain relievers as a result of a chronic ailment. However, the body develops used to these drugs with time. They grow less useful and may eventually cease to function. This means you'll probably need to take more pain relievers to achieve the same degree of relief. Pain relievers can have a variety of negative effects. Some of them are even addicting. High dosages of pain relievers are rarely seen as beneficial. And, in many cases, they just do not function to alleviate your discomfort.

Who should pursue IV pain relief therapy?

This form of treatment can help a lot of people. For example, if you have persistent pain from a car accident or back injury that isn't alleviated by standard care, IV therapy may be beneficial. Anyone suffering from disease-related discomfort, such as cancer or fibromyalgia, is likely to benefit from IV treatment. It can also be used to help avoid long-term discomfort. If you have an injury that isn't healing quickly or you want to make sure it heals completely, IV treatment can be quite beneficial. It may even aid in the prevention of chronic pain.

Getting IV treatment might be one of the finest things you can do for yourself - here's how to get started. At Balance Hormone Center, we work with you to create an IV therapy treatment plan that meets your specific needs. Our therapy choices are broad and can help with chronic pain management.

Chapter 4: Building Resilience with IV Therapy

Intravenous (IV) therapy has emerged as a potent technique for enhancing geriatric wellbeing and resilience. It is a living link between contemporary medical knowledge and the specific demands of the aging population. As we examine the notion of Building Resilience with IV Therapy, we will go on a journey to see how this medical wonder may improve not only the physical but also the emotional and mental well-being of seniors.

IV Therapy's Role in Senior Wellness

Aging is a normal and unavoidable process, but it frequently brings with it a set of obstacles that can have a negative influence on a senior's overall quality of life. Physical problems, lowered immune function, cognitive changes, and emotional pressures are among the obstacles. IV therapy has evolved as a holistic strategy to treating these issues and cultivating resilience in elders.

A. Physical Stability

1. IV Therapy for Prevention

Preventative approaches are one of the most important ways IV Therapy builds physical resilience in seniors. IV Therapy can help elderly maintain their health by correcting vitamin shortages, increasing immunological function, and enhancing overall vigor. This proactive approach can help to improve physical resilience by giving the body the building blocks it requires to function properly.

2. Chronic Disease Management

Diabetes, heart disease, and arthritis are all common chronic health issues among seniors. These disorders can have a significant influence on one's physical health and quality of life. IV therapy can supplement standard therapies by delivering focused symptom alleviation, increasing hydration, and promoting overall health. This strategy not only aids in the management of many chronic illnesses, but it also promotes physical resilience by minimizing the burden of sickness.

B. Emotional and mental fortitude

1. The Mind-Body Relationship

Resilience isn't only a physical trait; it's also strongly linked to mental and emotional well-being. IV Therapy acknowledges the deep relationship between the mind and the body. When elders receive IV treatments that relieve physical discomfort or address underlying health conditions, their mental state frequently improves significantly. Reduced pain, higher energy, and better general health can all lead to less stress, worry, and sadness, all of which contribute to emotional resilience.

2. Improving Cognitive Performance

Cognitive changes are a significant source of anxiety among the elderly. Dementia and moderate cognitive impairment can have an influence on memory, thinking, and decision-making. IV therapy, especially when used to treat vitamin shortages or supply neuroprotective chemicals, may improve cognitive performance. This not only promotes cognitive resilience but also improves emotional well-being.

IV Therapy as a Holistic Senior Wellness Approach

One of IV Therapy's primary characteristics in fostering resilience in seniors is its comprehensive approach to wellbeing. Unlike certain medical procedures, IV Therapy acknowledges that seniors are complex creatures with multiple needs.

A. Customized Care

IV therapy can be adjusted to each senior's specific needs. Healthcare providers evaluate the patient's health state, medical history, and particular concerns before delivering IV therapies.

This tailored approach guarantees that elders receive the most suitable and effective therapies to boost their resilience and well-being.

B. All-Inclusive Assistance

Seniors frequently suffer a variety of health issues, ranging from physical problems to mental burdens. IV Therapy gives complete help by addressing these issues holistically. IV Therapy may be a flexible tool in the senior wellness toolkit, whether it's used to relieve pain, increase immune function, or promote mental well-being.

V. Real-Life Resilience Stories

The influence of IV Therapy on resilience in seniors is not only theoretical; it can be seen in the real-life accounts of those who have benefited from it. Let's look at some intriguing examples:

A. Jane's Physical Resilience Journey

Jane, 72, has been suffering from rheumatoid arthritis for some years. Her condition's discomfort and joint stiffness had begun to impair her physical resiliency and general quality of life. Traditional drugs offered some comfort, but the side effects were difficult to bear.

Jane investigated IV Therapy as an adjuvant to her arthritis therapy after her doctor recommended it. Anti-inflammatory drugs and minerals known to enhance joint health were added in the IV infusions. Jane saw a significant improvement in her pain and movement over time. She was able to resume physical hobbies she had previously abandoned, such as gardening and going on walks with her friends. This physical toughness not only improved her everyday life, but it also improved her emotional well-being since she felt more connected to the things and people she enjoyed.

Cognitive Resilience of B. John

John, a retired teacher of 80, has noticed slight alterations in his memory and cognitive performance. He was anxious about the likelihood of dementia because his mother had suffered from it in her older years.

A full evaluation was ordered by John's healthcare practitioner, which found minor cognitive impairment. Along with cognitive exercises and lifestyle changes, John's healthcare team recommended IV Therapy as part of his treatment strategy. The IV therapy contained nutrition and neuroprotective chemicals.

John's cognitive performance improved over time, and he reported increases in his memory and clarity of reasoning. This cognitive endurance enabled him to pursue his interests, such as reading and writing. It also helped him with his emotional resilience by reducing the worry and panic that typically accompany cognitive loss.

Safety and Precautions

While IV Therapy has significant advantages for elder wellbeing and resilience, it is critical to address safety concerns.

A. Potential Hazards

IV Therapy, like any medical practice, has possible dangers. Infection at the injection site, vein irritation, allergic responses to the medicines injected, and problems connected to the puncture itself are among the hazards. Seniors, in particular, may have distinct risk factors, such as weakened immune systems or brittle veins, that must be carefully evaluated.

B. Ensured Security

Several precautions must be taken to protect the safety of elders receiving IV therapy:

1. Qualified Practitioners: IV Therapy should only be provided by trained and experienced healthcare professionals. This reduces the risk of problems and ensures that therapies are customized to the unique needs of the individual.

2. tight Protocol Adherence: During IV Therapy sessions, healthcare professionals should follow tight procedures for infection control, sterile technique, and monitoring. This involves employing aseptic practices when placing the IV catheter, keeping a sterile area, and monitoring the patient's vital signs and overall well-being during the treatment.

3. Patient Evaluation: Before beginning IV Therapy, a comprehensive patient evaluation is required. This evaluation should involve a look at the patient's medical history, current medicines, allergies, and any underlying health issues. Factors that may raise the risk of problems, such as a history of clotting disorders or reduced immunological function, should be given special consideration.

4. Vein Selection: Choosing a suitable vein for IV insertion is crucial, particularly in seniors with fragile or damaged veins. Healthcare personnel should thoroughly assess the veins, taking into account criteria like size, accessibility, and the patient's comfort.

5. Hydration Checking: Seniors are more prone to fluid imbalances. As a result, careful monitoring of hydration status is essential throughout IV therapy. The pace and amount of IV fluids should be adjusted based on the patient's particular needs and reaction.

6. Allergy and medicine History: Because seniors have a longer history of medicine usage, they are more likely to develop allergies or drug interactions. To detect any possible difficulties, healthcare practitioners should extensively analyze the patient's drug history and choose IV therapy accordingly.

7. Documentation: Complete and accurate documentation of IV Therapy sessions is critical for patient safety. This involves keeping track of the kind and volume of IV fluids given, the drugs given, vital signs, the state of the insertion site, and any adverse reactions or problems.

8. Informed Consent: Seniors should be given complete information about the IV Therapy treatment, including its advantages, hazards, and alternatives. Before beginning therapy, acquire informed consent to verify that the patient completely knows and consents to the process.

C. The Importance of Medical Monitoring

IV Therapy should be administered to seniors, especially those with complicated medical histories or numerous health issues, under the supervision of a skilled healthcare professional. This guarantees that any unanticipated issues are handled quickly and that the treatment plan may be altered as needed.

Seniors should also be encouraged to communicate openly with their healthcare provider during the IV Therapy procedure. Any concerns or changes in their health state should be communicated to their healthcare practitioner as soon as possible in order to support a proactive and tailored approach to care.

IV Therapy's Future in Senior Healthcare

The healthcare landscape is always changing, and IV Therapy is no exception. We may expect some new advancements in the field of IV Therapy for Seniors as medical research develops and our understanding of senior health increases.

A. Current Research and Development

IV Therapy advantages and uses are still being researched. Scientists are investigating new IV solution formulations, novel intravenous medicines, and novel delivery systems to improve the efficacy and safety of IV therapy for seniors. This steady progress bodes well for broadening the variety of illnesses that can be adequately treated with IV Therapy.

B. Seniors' Individualized Therapies

We should expect the creation of personalized IV Therapy regimens suited to certain age-related illnesses as we obtain a better knowledge of the distinct health demands of elders. These protocols may target concerns including cognitive decline, immunological support, and pain management with great accuracy, providing elders with increasingly individualized and effective treatment.

The use of IV Therapy in elder healthcare, on the other hand, should always be addressed with a dedication to safety and tailored care. Healthcare providers and seniors themselves play critical responsibilities in ensuring that

IV Therapy is used safely and effectively as part of a complete wellness approach.

Looking ahead, the growth of IV Therapy in elder healthcare promises to broaden the frontiers of what is possible. Ongoing research and individualized therapies have the potential to open up even more chances for seniors to build and preserve resilience, allowing them to live their golden years to the fullest with energy, strength, and emotional well-being.

www.ingramcontent.com/pod-product-compliance
Lightning Source LLC
Chambersburg PA
CBHW062326290526
45794CB00005B/1916